HEALTHY MEAL PREP COOKBOOK

Quick and Delicious Recipes for Balanced Living

Abbey Thompson

Copyright © 2024 by [Abbey Thompson]

TABLE OF CONTENT

DAILY MEAL REMARK

INTRODUCTION

Welcome to the "Healthy Meal Prep Cookbook"! Whether you're a busy professional, a parent juggling multiple responsibilities, or simply someone who wants to take control of their diet, meal prepping can be a game-changer. This cookbook is designed to guide you through the ins and outs of meal prep, ensuring you have delicious, nutritious meals ready to go, no matter how hectic your schedule may be.

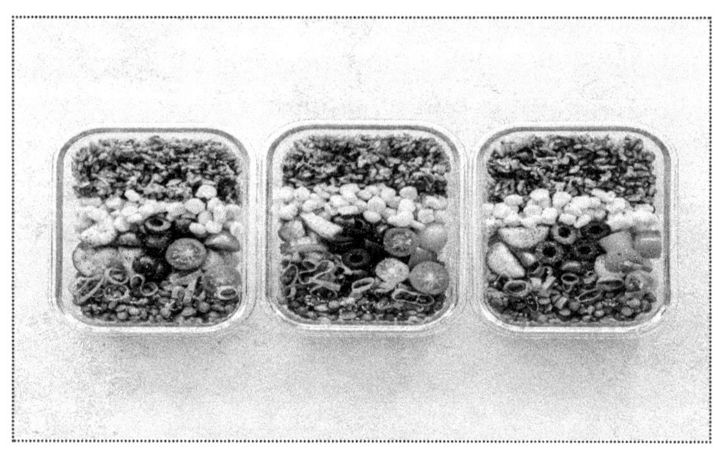

CHAPTER ONE

The Benefits of Meal Prepping

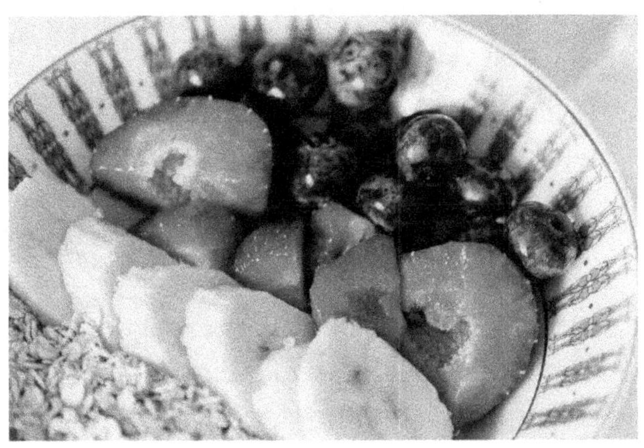

Meal prepping isn't just a trend—it's a lifestyle change that offers numerous benefits:

1. Saves Time: By setting aside a few hours once a week to prepare your meals, you can significantly reduce the time spent cooking each day. No more last-minute scrambles to put together a healthy dinner or grabbing unhealthy takeout because you're too tired to cook.

2. Saves Money: Planning your meals in advance helps you avoid impulse buys and reduces food waste. When you know exactly what you need, you can buy in bulk and take advantage of sales, stretching your grocery budget further.

3. Promotes Healthy Eating: With pre-prepared meals ready to go, you're less likely to reach for unhealthy snacks or fast food. Meal prepping allows you to control the ingredients and portion sizes, helping you stay on track with your health and fitness goals.

4. Reduces Stress: Knowing that you have a fridge full of ready-to-eat meals can reduce the stress of daily meal planning and cooking. It gives you more time to focus on other important aspects of your life.

5. Supports Weight Management: When your meals are planned and portioned in advance, it's easier to manage calorie intake and make healthier choices, aiding in weight loss or maintenance.

Essential Tools and Equipment

To get started with meal prepping, you'll need a few key tools and equipment. Here's a list of essentials that will make your meal prep journey smoother and more efficient:

-Containers: Invest in high-quality, reusable containers in various sizes. Look for containers that are microwave-safe, dishwasher-safe, and have leak-proof lids.

- **Measuring Cups and Spoons:** Accurate measurements are crucial for portion control and following recipes co

-**Cutting Boards and Knives:** Sharp knives and sturdy cutting boards are essential for efficient chopping and slicing.

- **Sheet Pans and Baking Dishes:** These are perfect for preparing large batches of roasted vegetables, baked proteins, and casseroles.

- **Slow Cooker or Instant Pot:** These appliances are great for hands-off cooking, allowing you to prepare large quantities of food with minimal effort.

- **Blender or Food Processor:** Useful for making smoothies, soups, sauces, and even chopping vegetables quickly.

Tips for Efficient Meal Prep

To make the most of your meal prep sessions, consider these tips:

1. Plan Ahead: Decide on your meals for the week and create a detailed shopping list. Planning ahead will help you stay organized and ensure that you have all the ingredients you need for your meal.

2. Batch Cooking: Prepare large quantities of staple ingredients like grains, proteins, and vegetables. These can be mixed and matched throughout the week to create different meals.

3. Use Versatile Ingredients: Choose ingredients that can be used in multiple recipes. For example, roasted chicken can be used in salads, wraps, and grain bowls.

4. Stay Organized: Label your containers with the meal and date. This helps you keep track of what needs to be eaten first and prevents food from going to waste.

5. Keep it Simple: Start with a few simple recipes and gradually add more as you become more comfortable with the process. Overcomplicating things can lead to burnout.

Meal prepping is a journey, and like any journey, it gets easier with practice. This cookbook is here to provide you with the knowledge, tools, and recipes you need to make healthy meals prepping a seamless part of your life. So, let's get started on the path to healthier, stress-free.

CHAPTER TWO

Nutritional Fundamentals

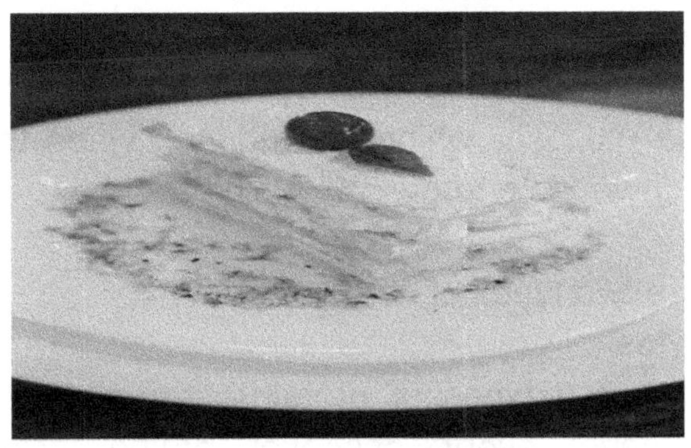

Basics of Nutrition

To prepare nutritious, well-balanced meals that nourish your body and enhance your general wellbeing, it is essential to understand nutrition. You will learn the fundamentals of macronutrients, micronutrients, and how to balance your diet for the best possible health in this chapter.

Understanding Macronutrients

The nutrients your body needs in large quantities to maintain biological processes and produce energy are known as macronutrients. Three primary categories of macronutrients exist:

1.Carbohydrates:
Purpose
Carbohydrates are the body's source of energy. Your cells use glucose, which is produced when they are broken down, as energy.
Types
There are two types of carbohydrates
Categories
There are two types of proteins: complete proteins (which have every essential amino acid) and incomplete proteins (which lack one or more). All of the essential amino acids can be obtained by combining different plant proteins.
Sources: Dairy products, eggs, poultry, fish, legumes, nuts, seeds, and soy products.

3. Fats:
Purpose
Fats shield organs, offer a concentrated source of energy, promote cell growth, and aid in the absorption of several vitamins (A, D, E, and K).

Reduce your intake of trans and saturated fats and increase your intake of unsaturated fats.

Sources
Nuts, seeds, avocados, olive oil, fatty fish, and, in moderation, coconut oil.

Micronutrients: What's at Stake

Micronutrients are vitamins and minerals that are essential for overall health but are required by your body in lesser amounts:

1. Vitamins
 -Water-Soluble Vitamins: These consist of vitamins C and B. Since the body cannot store these vitamins, constant consumption is required.
-Vitamins that are soluble in fat: they include A, D, E, and K. Together with dietary lipids, they are absorbed and retained by the body.
Features
Promote the health of your bones, blood coagulation, energy production, immune system, and more.

2. Minerals:
Calcium, phosphorus, potassium, sodium, magnesium, and chloride are among the major minerals.

- Trace Minerals: These consist of iodine, iron, manganese, copper, zinc, and selenium.

- **Supports:** Enzyme activity, fluid balance, bone health, oxygen transfer, and more.

Keeping Your Diet in Balance for Optimal Health

To make sure your body gets all the vital elements it needs, a balanced diet consists of a variety of foods. The following advice can help you maintain a balanced diet:

1. Incorporate a Variety of Foods: To guarantee a wide range of nutrients, eat a variety of fruits, vegetables, whole grains, proteins, and healthy fats.

2. Portion Control: To prevent overindulging and preserve a healthy weight, pay attention to portion proportions. If necessary, use a food scale or measuring cups.

3. Equilibrium of Macronutrients: Try to incorporate all three (carbs, proteins, and fats) into each meal. This gives you long-lasting energy and keeps you feeling fulfilled.

4. Limit Processed Foods: Consume less high-sugar and processed foods. These frequently lack vital nutrients, which can lead to weight gain and other health problems.

5. Remain Hydrated: Throughout the day, sip lots of water. Drinking enough water is crucial for healthy digestion, absorption of nutrients, and general wellbeing.

Example of a Well-Balanced Meal Plan

The following two sample balanced meal plans will help you understand how to mix various foods to satisfy your nutritional needs:

Sample Day 1:

Breakfast: Greek yogurt with mixed berries, chia seeds, and a sprinkle of honey.

Lunch: Quinoa salad with black beans, cherry tomatoes, cucumber, avocado, and a lime vinaigrette.

Dinner: Carrot sticks with hummus, baked salmon along with roasted sweet potatoes and steamed broccoli.

Snack: Apple

Sample Day 2:

Breakfast: Overnight oats cooked with almond milk, topped with banana slices, walnuts, and a sprinkling of cinnamon.

Lunch: Whole grain wrap with grilled chicken, mixed greens, shredded carrots, and a tahini dressing.

Dinner: Soy-ginger stir-fried tofu with brown rice, bell peppers, and snap peas.

Snack: Pineapple chunks mixed with cottage cheese.

In summary

The foundation of healthy meal preparation is an understanding of nutrition principles. You can make meals that taste wonderful and benefit your overall health by adding a range of nutrient-dense foods and balancing your intake of macronutrients and micronutrients. You will discover a multitude of recipes and advice to assist you in implementing these dietary principles as you proceed through this cookbook.

CHAPTER THREE

Easy and Healthful Breakfast

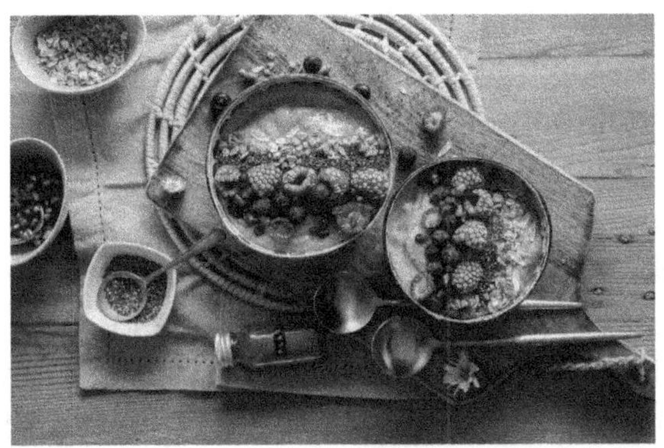

A healthy breakfast can help you establish the mood for the rest of the day. This chapter will cover a range of breakfast options that are simple to make ahead of time, so no matter how hectic your morning becomes, you can always start your day off well.

Recipes Smoothies Packed with Protein for Overnight Oats

A flexible and quick breakfast alternative, overnight oats can be tailored to your personal preferences. To help you get started, consider these delectable recipes:

1. Traditional Overnight Oats: Components

 - 1/2 cup almond milk (or any other type of   milk of your choice)
- 1/2 cup rolled oats
- 1/4 teaspoon vanilla extract
- 1 tablespoon chia seeds
- 1 tablespoon maple syrup
- Fresh fruit (banana slices, berries, etc.) for garnish

Guidelines
1. Place the oats, milk, chia seeds, maple syrup, vanilla essence in an airtight jar or mason jar.
2. Give it a good stir, cover it, and chill it for the night.
3. Before serving in the morning, give it a nice toss and sprinkle some fresh fruit on top.

2. Overnight Oats with Chocolate Peanut Butter: Ingredients
-Half a cup of rolled oats
- 1/2 cup of milk (optional)
- One tablespoon powdered cocoa
- One tablespoon of peanut butter
- One tablespoon chia seeds; - One tablespoon honey
- Shavings of dark chocolate for garnish (optional)

Guidelines
1. In a jar or other container, combine all ingredients except the chocolate shavings.
2. Store in the fridge for the night.

3. Give it a good stir in the morning, and if you like, garnish with shavings of dark chocolate.

To make Tropical Overnight Oats,
-combine 1/2 cup rolled oats and 1/2 cup coconut milk.
- 1/4 cup of shredded coconut
- 1/2 cup of sliced pineapple
- One teaspoon honey
- One tablespoon chia seeds

Guidelines
1. Fill a jar or other container with all the ingredients.
2. Give it a good stir, then chill for the night.
3. If desired, sprinkle with more pineapple and shredded coconut before serving cold.

Smoothies Packed with Protein

Smoothies are an excellent means of rapidly ingesting a large number of nutrients. Your mornings might be even easier if you prepare the smoothie packs ahead of time. Here are some recipes for protein-rich smoothies:

1.Green Power Smoothie
Ingredients
- Half a banana
- One cup spinach

-1/2 cup of frozen mango

-1 spoon of protein powder with vanilla flavor

- One cup of almond milk

-One-third cup chia seeds

Directions

1. Fill a blender with all the ingredients; process until smooth.

2. Transfer to a glass and start sipping right away.

2. Fruit Blast Smoothie:

Components

- 1/2 cup of mixed berries, including raspberries, blueberries, and strawberries; - 1/2 banana

- One cup of Greek yogurt

-1 tablespoon of flaxseed

- One cup water or your preferred milk

Guidelines

1. Fill a blender with all the ingredients, and process until smooth.

2. You can serve it right away or transfer it to a cup to go for a quick breakfast.

3. Chocolate Banana Protein Smoothie: - 1 banana as an ingredient

- One tablespoon powdered cocoa

- One spoon of chocolate-flavored protein powder

 - One cup of choice of milk

 - One tablespoon of almond butter

Guidelines

1. Purée every component until it's smooth.

2. Savor right away for a protein-packed, chocolate-flavored bread.

Premade Egg Muffins

A quick and easy method to have a high-protein breakfast on hand is to make egg muffins. Here are some dishes you should try:

1. Egg Muffins with Spinach and Feta: Ingredients

- Six big eggs

- 1/4 cup sliced red bell pepper

- 1/2 cup crumbled feta cheese

- 1 cup chopped fresh spinach

- Salt and pepper to taste

Guidelines

1. Oil a muffin tray and preheat the oven to 350°F (175°C).
2. Beat the eggs thoroughly in a bowl.
3. Add the bell pepper, spinach, feta, salt, and pepper.
4. Evenly fill the muffin cups with the egg mixture.
5. Bake the muffins for 20 to 25 minutes, or until they are slightly brown and firm.
6. Allow to cool before Taking Out of Tin. Keep chilled for a maximum of five days.

2. Egg Muffins with Ham and Cheese: Ingredients
- Six big eggs
- 1/2 cup chopped ham
- 1/2 cup of cheddar cheese, shredded
-Diced green onions, 1/4 cup
-To taste, add salt and pepper.

Guidelines
1. Oil a muffin tray and preheat the oven to 350°F (175°C).
2. In a bowl, whisk the eggs.
3. Gently stir in the ham, cheese, green onions, salt, and pepper.
4. Fill the muffin cups with the mixture.
5. Bake the muffins for 20 to 25 minutes, or until they are set.

6. Allow it to cool completely before you take it out of the tin. Keep chilled for a maximum of five days.

3. Egg Muffins with Veggies Packed:
Components:
  - Six big eggs
  -1/4 cup of tomatoes, diced
   - 1/4 cup sliced bell peppers; - 1/4 cup diced zucchini
  - 1/4 cup finely chopped onions
 - Half a cup of mozzarella cheese, shredded
  -To taste, add salt and pepper.

Guidelines
1. Oil a muffin tray and preheat the oven to 350°F (175°C).
2. In a bowl, whisk the eggs.
3. Add the cheese, salt, pepper, and veggies and stir.
4. Evenly distribute the mixture among the muffin liners.
5. Bake the muffins for 20 to 25 minutes, or until they are firm and have a hint of color.
6. Allow to cool before taking out of the tin. Keep chilled for a maximum of five days.

In summary

Making a healthy breakfast doesn't have to take a lot of time. These easy-to-make recipes for protein-rich smoothies, overnight oats, and egg muffins can help you start your day off well with little work. We'll go over lunch, supper, and snack meal prep ideas in the upcoming chapters to help you have a balanced diet all day.

CHAPTER FOUR

Lunch Preps

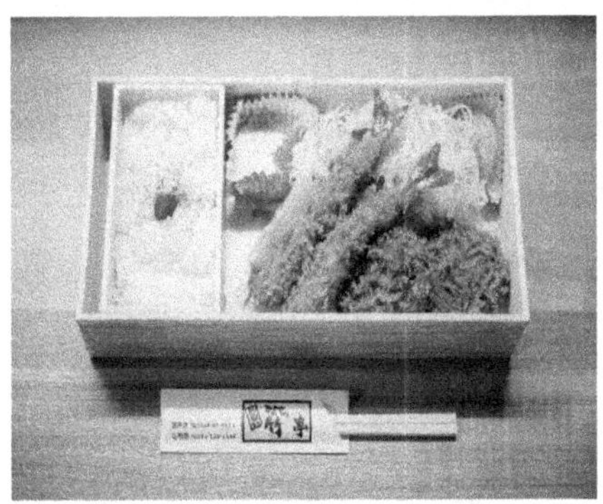

Eating a nutritious, easily portable lunch can significantly impact your ability to sustain your energy and work output during the day. This chapter will cover many lunch prep ideas that are tasty, nutrient-dense, and simple to make.

Well-Blended Grain Bowls

A healthy and adaptable lunch choice are grain bowls. Usually, they are made up of a base of grains, an assortment of vegetables, a source of protein, and a tasty dressing. To get you going, consider these suggestions:

1. Mediterranean Quinoa Bowl:
Ingredients:
-1 cup cooked quinoa -
1/2 cup halved cherry tomatoes
-1/2 cup diced cucumber
-1/4 cup thinly sliced red onion
-1/4 cup pitted and sliced Kalamata olives
-1/4 cup of feta cheese crumbles
-1/4 cup of hummus
-1 tablespoon of olive oil
-1 tablespoon of lemon juice
- To taste, add salt and pepper.

Guidelines

1. Distribute the cooked quinoa among meal preparation containers.

2. Add feta cheese, cherry tomatoes, cucumber, red onion, and olives on top.

3. Combine the lemon juice, olive oil, salt, and pepper in a small bowl.

4. Spoon the bowls with the dressing and top with a dollop of hummus.

5. Keep chilled for a maximum of four days.

2.Southwest Brown Rice Bowl are as follows:
Ingredients
-1 cup cooked brown rice;/
-1/2 cup rinsed and drained black beans-
1/2 cup corn kernels

-1/2 cup halved cherry tomatoes

- 1/4 cup diced red bell pepper

-1/4 cup shredded cheddar cheese

- 1/4 cup salsa.

- One sliced avocado

- One tablespoon lime juice

- One tablespoon chopped cilantro

- Toppings of salt and pepper

Guidelines

1. Fill meal prep containers with cooked brown rice.

2. Add cheddar cheese, bell pepper, cherry tomatoes, corn, and black beans on top.

3. Include a couple avocado slices and a teaspoon of salsa.

4. Add a lime juice drizzle and chopped cilantro on top.

5. Keep chilled for a maximum of four days.

3. **Farro Bowl with an Asian Flavor:**
Ingredients

 -1 cup cooked farro

-1/2 cup shelled edamame

-1/2 cup shredded carrots

- 1/4 cup chopped green onions

- 1/2 cup thinly sliced red cabbage

- 1/4 cup chopped peanuts

- One tablespoon of sesame seeds

-1/4 cup of homemade or store-bought sesame dressing

Guidelines

1. Distribute the cooked farro among the meal containers.
2. Add edamame, green onions, red cabbage, and shredded carrots on top.
3. Add sesame seeds and chopped peanuts on top.
4. Pour sesame dressing over.
5. Keep chilled for a maximum of four days.

Healthy Wraps and Sandwiches

Sandwiches and wraps are quick and simple to prepare, and they may be loaded with a range of nutritious ingredients. Here are some delectable choices:

1. Avocado and Turkey Wrap: Components
-One whole-wheat tortilla
- 1/4 cup mixed greens
- 1/2 sliced avocado
- 4 slices of deli turkey
- 1/4 cup of carrots, shredded
-A tablespoon of hummus.

Guidelines

1. Place the tortilla flat and cover it equally with hummus.
2. Arrange the shredded carrots, mixed greens, avocado, and turkey slices on top.

3. Tightly roll the tortilla, then cover with plastic wrap or foil.

4. Keep chilled for a maximum of three days.

2. Sandwich with Chickpea Salad: Ingredients
- 1 can of washed, drained chickpeas
- Two tablespoons of Greek yogurt
- One tablespoon lemon juice

- One tablespoon Dijon mustard
- Diced celery stalk
- Finely chopped 1/4 cup red onion
- Season with salt and pepper
- 4 slices whole grain bread
- Lettuce leaves

Guidelines
1. Using a fork, mash the chickpeas until they are chunky in a bowl.

2. Add the lemon juice, red onion, celery, Greek yogurt, and Dijon mustard.

3. To taste, add salt and pepper for seasoning.

4. Top two slices of bread with the chickpea mixture and garnish with lettuce leaves.

5. To assemble sandwiches, place the remaining bread slices on top.

6. Keep chilled for a maximum of three days.

3. Hummus and Veggie Wrap: Components
-One whole-wheat tortilla

- 1/4 cup of carrot shreds
- 1/4 cup of hummus
- 1/4 cup of sliced cucumber
- 1/4 cup chopped red bell pepper
- 1/4 cup of leaf spinach

Guidelines

1. Evenly cover the tortilla with hummus.

2. Arrange the bell pepper, spinach, cucumber, and shredded carrots on top.

3. Tightly roll the tortilla, then cover with plastic wrap or foil.

4. Keep chilled for a maximum of three days.

Maintain-Fresh Salads

Lunch options that are both nourishing and refreshing can include salads. You can prepare salads that will keep for several days with a little advance planning. Here are some suggestions:

1. Greek salad in a Mason Jar: Ingredients

-1/4 cup Greek dressing
- 1/2 cup halved cherry tomatoes
- 1/2 cup diced cucumber
- 1/4 cup thinly sliced red onion
- 1/4 cup pitted and sliced Kalamata olives
- Two cups of mixed greens
- 1/4 cup of crumbled feta cheese

Guidelines

1. Arrange the ingredients in a mason jar according to this order: Mixed greens, feta cheese, cherry tomatoes, cucumbers, red onions, olives, and Greek dressing.

2. Cover the jar and keep it in the fridge for a maximum of four days.

3. Shake the container to combine the ingredients and transfer into a bowl when ready to eat.

2. Chicken Caesar Salad:
Ingredients

- 2 cups chopped romaine lettuce
- 1/2 cup diced cooked chicken breast
- 1/4 cup halved cherry tomatoes
- 1/4 cup croutons
- 2 tablespoons grated Parmesan cheese
- 1/4 cup Caesar dressing

Instructions

1. Layer the romaine lettuce, chicken, cherry tomatoes, croutons, and Parmesan cheese in a meal prep container

2. Store the Caesar dressing in a separate small container

3. Keep it refrigerated for up to 3 days

4. Add the dressing to the salad and toss to mix.

3. Asian Style Chicken Salad: Components

- 2 cups of shredded Napa cabbage
- 1/2 cup of shredded cooked chicken breast
- 1/4 cup of sliced bell peppers
- 1/4 cup of shredded carrots
- 1/4 cup of green onions, sliced
-finely chopped peanuts
- 1/4 cup homemade or store-bought sesame dressing

Guidelines

1. Arrange the Napa cabbage, chicken, bell peppers, green onions, carrots, and peanuts in a meal prep container.
2. Keep the sesame dressing in a different, little jar.
3. Store in the fridge for a maximum of three days.
4. Add the dressing to the salad right before eating and toss to mix.

In summary

These simple meal prep ideas make lunchtime wholesome and hassle-free. You can make your noon meal exciting and fulfilling by choosing from a range of alternatives, such as fresh salads, nutritious wraps, and balanced grain bowls. We'll get into supper prep ideas in the upcoming chapter so you can have a healthy meal to cap off your day. Cheers to your preparation!

CHAPTER FIVE

Dinner Preps

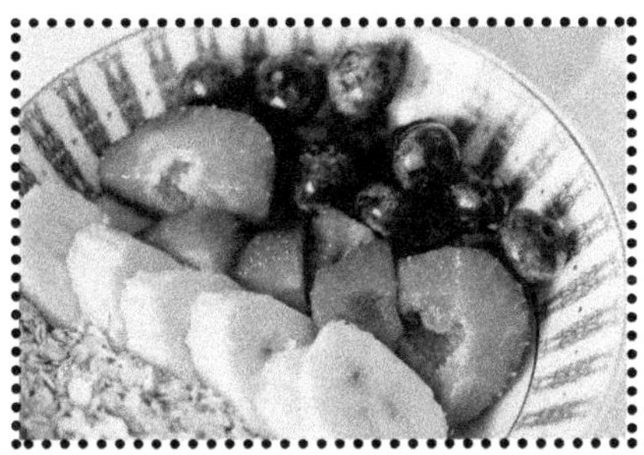

Since dinner is frequently the most looked forward to meal of the day, preparing it ahead of time may greatly enhance the leisure and enjoyment of your evenings. We'll look at a number of tasty and healthy supper prep options in this chapter, so you can make sure you finish your day with a filling meal.

Dinners in a Pan

Meal prep enthusiasts love one-pan dinners because they're easy to dish out for numerous meals and require little cleanup. Here are a few delectable choices:

1. Sheet Pan Chicken and Vegetables:
- Four skinless and boneless chicken breasts

- 1 cup baby carrots
- 2 cups halved baby potatoes
- 1 cup broccoli florets
- One teaspoon dried thyme
- Two tablespoons olive oil
- Two tablespoons balsamic vinegar
- One teaspoon garlic powder
-To taste, add salt and pepper.

Guidelines
1.Set the oven's temperature to 400°F, or 200°C.
2. Spread out on a sizable baking sheet the potatoes, broccoli, carrots, and chicken breasts.
3. Combine the olive oil, balsamic vinegar, garlic powder, thyme, salt, and pepper in a small bowl.
4. Pour the mixture over the veggies and chicken, turning to coat thoroughly.
5. Bake for 25 to 30 minutes, or until the veggies are soft and the chicken is cooked through.
6. Split and store in the refrigerator for up to 4 days in meal prep containers.

2. Asparagus with Lemon Garlic Shrimp:
Ingredients
- Two teaspoons of olive oil
- Two tablespoons of lemon juice

- One bunch of asparagus, chopped and trimmed into two-inch pieces
- One pound of big shrimp, skinned and deveined
- Three minced garlic cloves
- One teaspoon of oregano, dried
- Use pepper and salt to taste

Guidelines
Set the oven's temperature to 400°F, or 200°C.
2. Put the asparagus and shrimp in an arrangement on a wide baking sheet.
3. Combine the olive oil, lemon juice, oregano, garlic, salt, and pepper in a small bowl.
4. Pour the mixture over the asparagus and shrimp, stirring to coat thoroughly.
5. Bake for 10 to 12 minutes, or until the asparagus is soft and the shrimp are pink and opaque.
6. Transfer to meal prep containers and keep chilled for a maximum of three days.

3. Teriyaki Salmon and Vegetables:
Ingredients
- Four filets of salmon
-One cup of sliced bell peppers
- One cup sliced carrots

- One cup snow peas
– 1/4 cup sauce teriyaki
- One tablespoon of seeds, sesame
- 2 tablespoons green onions, chopped

Guidelines
1.Set the oven's temperature to 400°F, or 200°C.
2. Spread out on a big baking sheet the bell peppers, carrots, snow peas, and salmon filets.
3. Cover the fish and veggies with teriyaki sauce.
4. Garnish the top with sesame seeds.
5. Bake for 15 to 20 minutes, or until the veggies are soft and the salmon is cooked through.
6. Divide into meal prep containers and garnish with chopped green onions.
7.Keep refrigerated for up to three days.

Filling Soups & Stews

Comforting, easily prepared in big quantities, and ideal for meal preparation are soups and stews. Here are some delectable dish ideas:

1. Chicken and Vegetable Soup:
Ingredients
- One tablespoon of olive oil
- Diced onion
- 3 chopped garlic cloves
- 3 sliced carrots
- 3 sliced celery stalks

- 1 pound of diced chicken breast
– 6 cups chicken broth
– 1 cup chopped green beans
- 1 cup of kernel corn
-Diced tomatoes, one cup
- 1 teaspoon of dried thyme
- 1 teaspoon of dried basil
- To taste, salt and pepper

Guidelines

1. Heat the olive oil in a big saucepan over medium heat.
2. Add the garlic and onion, and cook until aromatic.
3. Include the chicken, carrots, and celery and simmer until the chicken is browned.
4. Add the green beans, corn, tomatoes, thyme, basil, salt, and pepper after adding the chicken stock.
5. Once the veggies are cooked, bring to a boil, lower the heat, and simmer for 20 to 25 minutes.
6. Split and store in the refrigerator for up to five days in meal prep containers.

2. Beef and Barley Stew

Ingredients

-1 tablespoon olive oil
-1 pound cubed beef stew meat
- 1 chopped onion

-Diced two cloves of garlic

-Sliced three carrots and three celery stalks

-Six cups beef broth

- one cup chopped tomatoes; one cup pearl barley

-One teaspoon of dried thyme

- one teaspoon of dry rosemary

-The right amount of salt and pepper

Directions

1. Place the olive oil in a big saucepan and heat it to medium.

2. Include the steak, letting it brown all around.

3. When the garlic and onion are aromatic, add them and sauté.

4. Add the tomatoes, beef broth, celery, carrots, barley, thyme, and rosemary along with the salt and pepper.

5. After bringing to a boil, lower the heat, and simmer the barley for 45 to 50 minutes, or until it becomes soft.

6. Transfer to meal prep containers and keep chilled for a maximum of five days.

3. Vegetable Lentil Stew:
Ingredients

- 1 tablespoon olive oil

- 1 chopped onion

-3 minced garlic cloves

- 3 sliced carrots

-3 sliced celery stalks

-1 cup dry lentils, washed

- One cup chopped tomatoes

- One teaspoon cumin

- One teaspoon paprika

- Six cups vegetable broth

- One-half teaspoon of turmeric

- Toppings of salt and pepper

Guidelines

1. Heat the olive oil in a big saucepan over medium heat.

2. Add the garlic and onion, and cook until aromatic.

3. Include the celery and carrots and simmer until just starting to soften.

4. Add the lentils, tomatoes, paprika, cumin, turmeric, salt, and pepper after stirring.

5. After bringing to a boil, lower the heat, and simmer the lentils for 30 to 35 minutes, or until they are soft.

6. Transfer to meal prep containers and keep chilled for a maximum of five days.

Reassuring casseroles

Because they are simple to prepare in big numbers and reheat nicely, casseroles are a traditional choice for meal prep. Here are some recipes for hearty casseroles:

Guidelines
1. Turn the oven on to 375°F, or 190°C.
2. Combine the chicken, broccoli, brown rice, cream of mushroom soup, cheddar cheese, Greek yogurt, garlic powder, onion powder, salt, and pepper in a big bowl.
3. Evenly distribute the ingredients in a baking dish.

4. Bake the casserole for 25 to 30 minutes, or until the cheese has melted and the dish is bubbling.
5. Split and store in the refrigerator for up to four days in meal prep containers.

2. **Vegetable Lasagna:**
Ingredients
Contains nine cooked lasagna noodles as an ingredient.
-One egg, two cups of ricotta cheese, one cup of shredded mozzarella cheese, and one cup of grated Parmesan cheese
- Two cups sauce marinara
- 2 cups chopped spinach
- 1 cup sliced mushrooms
- 1 sliced zucchini
-To taste, add salt and pepper.

Guidelines
1. Turn the oven on to 375°F, or 190°C.
2. Combine the spinach, ricotta cheese, egg, salt, and pepper in a bowl.
3. Line the bottom of a baking dish with a thin layer of marinara sauce.
4. Arrange three lasagna noodles on top of the sauce, then add mozzarella cheese, mushrooms, zucchini, and a third of the ricotta mixture.
5. Finish with a layer of noodles, sauce, and Parmesan cheese. Repeat layering two more times.
6. Bake, covered with foil, for 35 to 40 minutes.

In summary

By preparing your dinners ahead of time, you may enjoy wholesome, home-cooked meals without the stress of rushing to the kitchen. Dinner prep can turn your hectic nights into peaceful ones. You can guarantee your family has access to healthful and delectable dinners every night of the week by implementing one-pan meals, slow cooker recipes, and other prep-ahead supper ideas into your schedule. You'll have more opportunity to decompress and unwind after a demanding day with the time you save. Cheers to your preparation!

CHAPTER SIX

Snack Preps

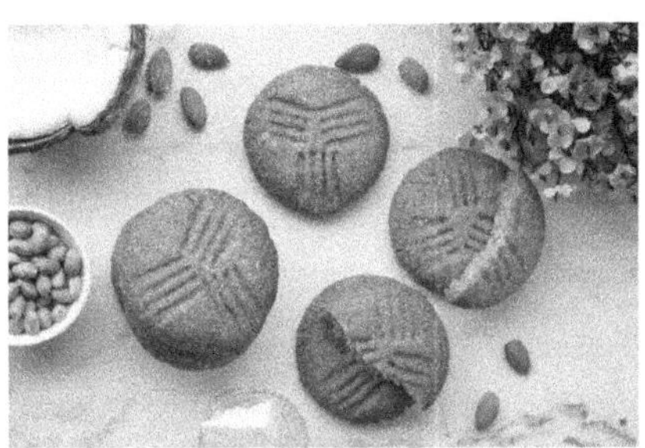

This chapter will walk you through a variety of snack prep ideas that are quick to prepare and ideal for on-the-go snacking. Energy Bites: Energy bites are a convenient and healthy snack option that can be customized to your liking. Try these delicious recipes.

1. Peanut Butter Energy Bites: Ingredients

-1 cup rolled oats

-1/2 cup peanut butter

-1/4 cup honey

-1/4 cup mini chocolate chips

- 1 tablespoon chia seeds

Guidelines

1. Place all the ingredients in a big bowl and stir until thoroughly mixed.

2. Form the mixture into tiny balls with a diameter of approximately an inch.

3. Transfer to a baking sheet covered with parchment paper, then chill for a minimum of half an hour.

4. For up to a week, keep in the refrigerator in an airtight container.

2. Coconut Almond Energy Bites:

Ingredients

-1/2 cup almond butter

- 1 cup rolled oats

- 1/4 cup of honey

- 1/4 cup of coconut shreds

- 1/4 cup of almonds

-1 tablespoon of flaxseed

Guidelines

1. In a large bowl, add all ingredients and stir until well blended.

2. Form the mixture into little balls and transfer to a baking sheet covered with parchment paper.

3. Transfer to an airtight container and refrigerate for a minimum of half an hour.

4. Keep chilled for a maximum of one week.

3. Chocolate Chip Cookie Dough Energy Bites:

Ingredients

-One cup of rolled oats

-half a cup of cashew butter

-one-fourth cup of honey

-one-fourth cup of micro chocolate chips

- One tablespoon of chia seeds

- One teaspoon of vanilla extract

Guidelines

1. In a large basin, thoroughly mix all ingredients together.

2. Using a baking sheet lined with parchment paper, form the mixture into tiny balls.

3. Allow it cool for a minimum of half an hour in the fridge.

4. For up to a week, keep in the refrigerator in an airtight container.

Dips and Veggie Packs

Snacking healthfully may be made simple and pleasurable by repackaging veggies with a delicious dip. Veggie and dip pack options include the following:

1. Hummus and Carrots:
Ingredients
- One cup of homemade or store-bought hummus
-two cups baby carrots

Guidelines
1. Scoop baby carrots into separate snack-sized jars.
2. Transfer hummus into little dip receptacles.

3. Combine the hummus and carrots for a simple and fast snack.
4. Keep chilled for a maximum of five days.

2. Celery and Peanut Butter:
Ingredients
- Two cups of carrot sticks
- Half a cup of peanut butter

Guidelines
1. Slice celery sticks into small pieces for snacking.
2. Transfer peanut butter into little dip receptacles.
3. Combine the peanut butter and celery for a wholesome snack.
4. Keep chilled for a maximum of five days.

3. Guacamole with Bell Peppers: Ingredients
- Two cups of bell peppers, sliced (any color)
A   - One cup of guacamole, handmade or from the store

Guidelines
1. Scoop out bell pepper slices and place them in separate snack-sized containers.
2. Divide the guacamole into little dip receptacles.
3. For a cool snack, combine the guacamole and bell peppers.
4. Keep chilled for a maximum of three days.

Mixtures of Fruit and Nuts

When fruits and nuts are combined, you may make a filling, healthy snack that's portable and simple to prepare. Here are a few combination ideas.

1.Tropical Trail Mix:
Ingredients
- 1/2 cup dried pineapple
-1/2 cup dry mango
- One-half cup coconut crisps
- One cup cashews
- One-half cup almonds

Guidelines
1. In a large bowl, combine all ingredients.
2. Split into separate bags or containers the size of snacks.
3. For up to two weeks, store at room temperature.

2. Berries and Nuts Mix:
Ingredients
- 1/2 cup dried cranberries
-50% dried blueberries
- 1/2 cup pecans
- 1/2 cup dark chocolate chips
- 1 cup walnuts

Guidelines

1. Put all the ingredients into a big basin and stir thoroughly.

2. Portion into containers or bags the size of snacks.

3. For up to two weeks, store at room temperature.

3. Apple Cinnamon Nut Mix:
Ingredients

- Selected apple slices, one cup
- 1/2 cup almonds with cinnamon
- Half a cup of raisins
- 1/2 cup of pumpkin seeds

Guidelines

1. In a large bowl, combine all ingredients.

2. Split into separate bags or containers the size of snacks.

3. For up to two weeks, store at room temperature.

Yogurt Confections

Parfaits made with yogurt are a tasty and nourishing pre-made snack. The following are some parfait suggestions:

1. Yogurt Parfait with Berries: Ingredients

- One cup of Greek yogurt
-1/2 cup of mixed berries, including raspberries, blueberries, and strawberries - 1/4 cup of granola
- One spoonful of honey

Guidelines

1. Arrange the mixed berries, granola, and Greek yogurt in a mason jar or other airtight container.
2. Pour some honey over it.
3. Keep chilled for a maximum of three days.

2. Yogurt Parfait with Tropical: Ingredients

- One cup of Greek yogurt
- 1/4 cup of shredded coconut
- 1/2 cup of chopped pineapple
- 1/2 cup of diced mango

Guidelines

1.Arrange the shredded coconut, pineapple, mango, and Greek yogurt in an airtight jar or mason jar.
2. Keep chilled for a maximum of three days.

3. Parfait with Apple Cinnamon Yogurt: Components

- One cup of Greek yogurt
- 1/2 cup of apple slices
- One teaspoon of cinnamon
- 1/4 cup of granola

Guidelines

First, arrange the Greek yogurt, chopped apples, granola, and a dash of cinnamon in an airtight jar or mason jar.

2. Keep chilled for a maximum of three days.

In summary

With these ideas for snack prep, you'll always have a wholesome and filling choice on hand, which will help you stay energized and resist cravings all day. These snacks are tasty and nourishing, ranging from veggie packs and energy bites to yogurt parfaits and fruit and nut mixtures. We'll look at dessert prep ideas in the next chapter so you can indulge in sweets without sacrificing your healthy eating objectives. Chewing pleasure!

CHAPTER SEVEN

Dessert Preps

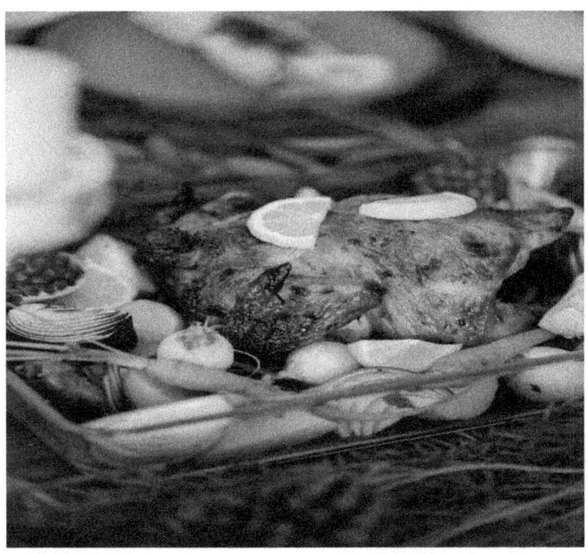

Who says you can't lead a healthy lifestyle and still enjoy decadent desserts? If you prepare desserts ahead of time, you'll always have wholesome, filling treats on hand for when your sugar craving strikes. You're going to find lots of delicious, guilt-free dessert prep ideas in this chapter.

Nutritious Baked Goods

In addition to being a satisfying treat, baked goods can be nutritious with a few nutritious modifications. Here are some suggestions for nutritious baked goods:

Banana Oat Muffins:
Ingredients
-2 ripe, mashed bananas
- 1/4 cup honey
- 1/4 cup melted coconut oil
- 2 eggs
- 1 1/2 cups rolled oats
- 1 teaspoon baking powder
- 1 teaspoon vanilla extract
- Half a teaspoon of baking soda
- 1/4 teaspoon salt
- 1/2 teaspoon cinnamon

Guidelines
1. Grease a muffin tin with paper liners and preheat the oven to 350°F (175°C).
2. Put the mashed bananas, eggs, coconut oil, honey, and vanilla extract in a big bowl.
3. Combine the rolled oats, baking soda, baking powder, cinnamon, and salt in a different bowl.
4. Stir just until fully combined after adding the dry ingredients to the wet ones.

5. Evenly distribute the batter among the muffin tins.

6. Bake the cake for twenty to twenty-five minutes, or until a toothpick inserted in the center comes out clean.

7. Let cool fully before storing for up to five days in an airtight container.

2. Brownies Made with Almond Flour: Ingredients:

-1 cup almond flour

- 1/4 cup cocoa powder

- Half a teaspoon of baking soda

- 1/4 teaspoon salt

- 1/2 cup chips made of dark chocolate

- 1/4 cup melted coconut oil

- 1/4 cup honey

- Two eggs

- One tsp of vanilla extract

Guidelines

1. Preheat the oven to 350°F (175°C), and place parchment paper inside an 8-by-8-inch baking pan.

2. Combine almond flour, baking soda, cocoa powder, and salt in a bowl.

3. Combine the coconut oil and dark chocolate chipsin a different bowl and melt them.

4. Thoroughly combine the melted chocolate mixture with the eggs, honey, and vanilla extract.

5. Mix the dry and wet ingredients together, stirring to ensure smoothness.

6. Evenly distribute the batter into the baking pan that has been prepared.

7. Bake for 20-25 minutes, or until a toothpick inserted in the center emerges clean.

8. Let it cool fully before slicing it into squares. For up to five days, store in an airtight container.

3. Pumpkin Spice Cookies:
Ingredients
- 1 cup canned pureed pumpkin
-1/2 cup honey; 1/4 cup melted coconut oil; 1 egg
- Two cups almond flour
- One teaspoon vanilla extract
- One tsp baking powder
- Half a teaspoon of baking soda
- 1/2 teaspoon nutmeg
- 1 teaspoon cinnamon
- 1/4 teaspoon of salt
- 1/4 teaspoon of cloves

Guidelines
Preheat the oven to 350°F (175°C), and place parchment paper on a baking sheet.

2. Put the pureed pumpkin, honey, coconut oil, egg, and vanilla extract in a big bowl.

3. Combine almond flour, baking soda, nutmeg, cloves, cinnamon, and salt in a different bowl.

4. Combine the dry ingredients with the wet ingredients, stirring to fully blend.

5. Spoon dough onto the baking sheet that has been prepared, pressing it down slightly.

6. Bake for ten to twelve minutes, or until the sides are browned.

7. Let cool fully before storing for up to five days in an airtight container.

No-Bake Sweets

No-bake desserts are an easy and nutritious dessert option because they're quick to make and store well in the refrigerator or freezer. Try these dishes:

1. Chocolate Avocado Pudding: Ingredients

-1/4 cup cocoa powder

-2 ripe avocados

- 1/4 cup almond milk

- 1/4 cup honey

- One tsp of vanilla extract

Guidelines

1. Put avocados, cocoa powder, honey, almond milk, and vanilla extract in a food processor or blender.

2. Blend until creamy and smooth.

3. Transfer the pudding into separate serving dishes using a spoon.

4. Before serving, let the food cool in the refrigerator for at least half an hour.

5. Keep chilled for a maximum of three days.

2. Peanut Butter Chocolate Chip Balls:

Ingredients:

-1/2 cup peanut butter

-1 cup rolled oats

- 1/4 cup mini chocolate chips

- 1/4 cup honey

- One tsp of vanilla extract

Guidelines

1. Place all the ingredients in a big bowl and stir until thoroughly mixed.

2. Form the mixture into tiny balls with a diameter of about an inch.

3. Transfer to a baking sheet covered with parchment paper, then chill for a minimum of half an hour.

4. For up to a week, keep in the refrigerator in an airtight container.

3.Coconut Macaroons:

Ingredients

-2 cups of shredded coconut

- 1/2 cup almond flour
- 1/4 cup honey
- 1/4 cup melted coconut oil
- 1/4 teaspoon salt
- 1/4 teaspoon vanilla extract

Guidelines

1. Combine the chopped coconut, almond flour, honey, coconut oil, vanilla extract, and salt in a big bowl.

2. Blend until thoroughly blended.

3. Transfer the mixture by spoonfuls onto a parchment paper-lined baking sheet.

4. Create little mounds by pressing the mixture together.

5. To set, refrigerate for a minimum of 30 minutes.

6. Keep refrigerated in an airtight container for up to one week.

Ice Cream Confectionery

A healthy and refreshing way to indulge your sweet tooth is with frozen desserts. Here are some ideas for frozen treats:

1. Popsicles with Berry Yogurt: Ingredients
- Two cups of Greek yogurt

- One cup of mixed berries, comprising raspberries, blueberries, and strawberries
– Two tablespoons of honey

Guidelines

1. Place Greek yogurt, mixed berries, and honey in a blender.
2. Process until smooth.
3. Transfer the blend into popsicle molds and place sticks inside.
4. Freeze until solid, or for at least 4 hours.
5. For up to two months, store in the freezer.

2. Mango Coconut Ice Cream:
Ingredients

- 2 cups frozen mango chunks
- 1 cup coconut milk
-2 tablespoons honey
-and 1 teaspoon vanilla extract

Instructions

1. Put the frozen mango, coconut milk, honey, and vanilla extract in a blender.
2. Blend until creamy and smooth.
3. Transfer the mixture to a container that can be frozen, and leave it there for at least four hours.
4. For up to two months, store in the freezer.

3. Chocolate Banana Bites:

Ingredients

- Two sliced bananas
- Half a cup of chips, dark chocolate
- One tablespoon of coconut oil

Guidelines

1. Parchment paper should be spread over the baking sheet.

2. Place the slices of banana on the baking sheet.

3. Combine the dark chocolate chips and coconut oil in a bowl that is safe to use in the microwave. Stir until smooth.

4. Coat every slice of banana completely by dipping it into the melted chocolate.

5. Return the banana slices covered in chocolate to the baking sheet lined with parchment.

6. Freeze until solid, or for at least two hours.

Aw7. Keep in the freezer in an airtight container for up to two months.

In summary

You can enjoy tasty and healthful sweet treats with these ideas for dessert prep. These recipes, which range from refreshing frozen desserts to baked goods and no-bake treats, will satiate your cravings without sacrificing your healthy eating objectives. To help you stay organized and get the most out of your meal prep efforts, we'll go over how to effectively plan your weekly meal prep in the upcoming chapter. Cheers to a happy indulgence!

CHAPTER EIGHT

Weekly Meal Planning

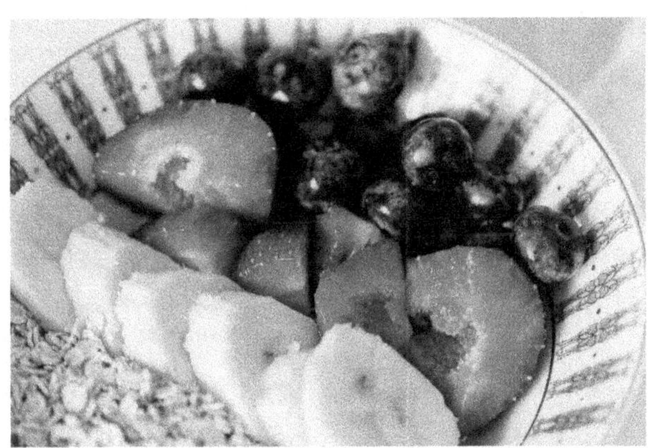

A thoughtful plan is the first step towards effective meal prep. You can ensure you have a balanced diet, save time, and cut down on food waste by planning your meals for the week. This chapter will walk you through the process of organizing your weekly menu, from making a shopping list and meal plan to cooking and storing your food.

Planning Your Meals

Making a meal plan is the first step in weekly meal prep. This is how to begin:

1.Evaluate Your Timetable: Examine your weekly schedule on the calendar. Note any days when you have a lot on your plate or when you won't be home for dinner. This will assist you in figuring out how many meals require preparation and which ones can be finished quickly.

2. Pick Your Recipes: Make a range of breakfast, lunch, dinner, snack, and dessert recipes. To make sure your mix of flavors and nutrients is well-balanced, think about utilizing recipes from earlier chapters.

3. Maintain a Nutrient Balance: Make sure that every meal includes an appropriate amount of protein, carbs, and healthy fats. To make sure you get a range of vitamins and minerals, include a variety of fruits and vegetables in your diet.

4. Make a Leftovers Plan: Include recipes that make leftovers. You'll be able to prepare fewer dishes and save time as a result of this.

5. Put It in Writing: Make a weekly meal plan template on paper or in digital format. Every day of the week, jot down the meals and snacks you eat. Keeping organized and identifying any gaps or redundancies will be made easier with the aid of this visual representation.

Putting Together a Purchase List

Making a thorough shopping list comes next after you have your meal plan. As follows:

1. List every ingredient: Make a list of all the ingredients you'll need by going through each recipe. Remember to take stock of what you already have by opening your pantry, refrigerator, and freezer.

2. Sort by Category: Assemble the ingredients into categories (such as produce, dairy, meat, and pantry essentials). This will increase the effectiveness of your shopping trip and guarantee that you don't miss anything.

3. Take Quantities into Account: Make a note of the amounts required for each ingredient to prevent purchasing too much or too little. If you intend to double a recipe or save some for later, then modify the amounts appropriately.

4. Add Non-Food Items: Don't forget to include any non-food items you may require, like freezer bags, aluminum foil, or storage containers.

5. Examine Sales and Coupons: Visit your neighborhood grocery store to see if there are any sales, discounts, or coupons. You can stay within your budget and save money by doing this:

Getting Your Meals Ready

It's time to prepare your meals now that you have your ingredients. Here are some pointers to make the procedure enjoyable and effective.

1. Set Aside Time: Decide on a day and time in advance to prepare meals. Weekends and evenings are often the most productive times for people. Give yourself a few hours to complete everything.

2. Gather Your Supplies: Ensure that you have all of the cutlery and saucepans, measuring cups, mixing bowls, cutting boards, knives, and storage containers that you'll need.

3. Prepare in Bulk: Commence with the jobs that take the longest, like roasting veggies or cooking grains. You can chop veggies, marinate proteins, or combine ingredients for other recipes while those are cooking.

4. Label and Store: After your meals are prepared, divide them into serving sizes and mark the contents and date on the container. Meals can be kept in the freezer or refrigerator, depending on when you want to eat them.

5. Keep It Clean: To keep your workspace organized and to make cleanup easier at the end, clean as you go. Clean surfaces, wash dishes, and take out the trash on a regular basis.

Meal Preservation and Reheating

To keep your prepared meals safe and of high quality, you must store and reheat them properly. What you should know is as follows:

1. Storage Containers: To keep your food fresh, use airtight containers. While BPA-free plastic containers are lightweight and practical, glass containers are excellent for reheating and environmentally friendly.

2. Labeling: To help you keep track of what needs to be eaten first and prevent any mystery meals, label each container with the contents and the date.

3. Refrigerating: If you intend to consume prepared meals within three to four days, keep them refrigerated. Freeze meals to maintain freshness and stop spoiling for extended storage.

4. Freezing: Be sure to allow room for expansion at the top of the container when freezing meals. Foods that freeze well include stews, casseroles, and soups.

5. Reheating: To guarantee that food is safe to eat, thoroughly reheat meals to an internal temperature of

165°F (74°C). Depending on what you're eating, use the oven, stovetop, or microwave.

6. Thawing: Use your microwave's defrost option or leave frozen meals in the fridge for the entire night to thaw. Steer clear of thawing at room temperature to stop the growth of bacteria.

Weekly Meal Plan Sample

Here's a sample weekly meal plan that uses recipes from this book to get you started:

Monday

Breakfast: Berries and Overnight Oats
Lunch: Mason Jar Greek Salad
Dinner: One-pan chicken with veggies
Snack: Energy Bites with peanut butter
Dessert: Chocolate Avocado Pudding

Tuesday

Breakfast: Egg Muffins with Veggie Filling
Lunch: Quinoa and black bean burrito bowls
Dinner: Slow-cooked stewed beef.
Snack: Hummus and carrots
Dessert: Brownies with almond flour

Wednesday

Breakfast: Smoothie packs
Lunch: Mason Jar Thai Noodle Salad
Dinner: Baked salmon served with asparagus and roasted potatoes.
Snack: Peanut butter and celery
Dessert: Berry Yogurt Popsicles

Thursday

Breakfast: Chia Pudding with Mango
Lunch: Mason Jar Greek Salad
Dinner: One-Pot Pasta Primavera
Snack: Bell Peppers and Guacamole
Dessert: Coconut Macaroons

Friday

Breakfast: Berries and Overnight Oats
Lunch: Quinoa and black bean burrito bowls
Dinner: Slow Cooker Chicken Chili
Snack: Peanut Butter Chocolate Chip Balls
Dessert: Pumpkin Spice Cookie

Saturday

Breakfast: Veggie Egg Muffins
Lunch: Mason Jar Thai Noodle Salad
Dinner: Baked salmon served with asparagus and roasted potatoes.
Snack: Hummus and carrots
Dessert: Mango Coconut Ice Cream

Sunday
Breakfast: Smoothie Packs
Lunch: Quinoa and black bean burrito bowls
Dinner: One-Pot Pasta Primavera
Snack: Peanut butter and celery
Dessert: Chocolate Banana Bites.

In summary

You can expedite your cooking process and enjoy a week of delectable, healthful meals without the daily hassle by organizing and preparing your meals in advance. This method decreases food waste, saves time and money, and assists you in maintaining your health goals. We'll look at some strategies for incorporating meal prep into your lifestyle in the upcoming chapter. Happy organizing!

CHAPTER NINE

Tips and Tricks for Sustainable Meal Prep

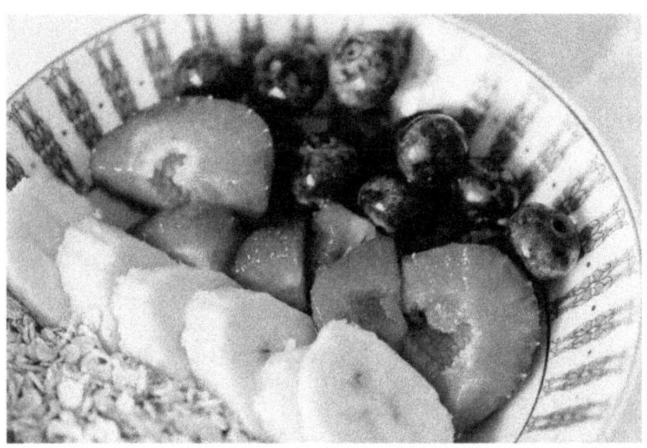

It takes planning, imagination, and flexibility to make meal preparation a fun and sustainable part of your life. You'll find helpful hints and techniques in this chapter to improve your meal prep routine, which will help you maintain consistency and motivation over time.

Effective Kitchen Arrangement

A well-organized kitchen is necessary for effective meal preparation. How to arrange your kitchen for success is as follows:

1. Designate Prep Areas: Set aside particular areas of your kitchen for food preparation, cooking, and storage. Your workflow will be streamlined as a result, increasing process efficiency.

2. Keep Necessities Handy: Keep frequently used items handy, such as measuring cups, mixing bowls, knives, and cutting boards. When preparing meals, this will cut down on frustration and save time.

3. Organize Pantry and Fridge: Use clear containers to allow for easy visibility and group similar items together to keep your pantry and refrigerator well-organized. To help you find what you need quickly, label shelves and containers.

Investing in high-quality kitchen tools can significantly impact the way you prepare meals. Think about making an investment in dependable storage containers, sturdy cutting boards, and sharp knives.

Cooking in Bulk

One excellent method to ensure you always have meals ready to go is to batch cook. Here are some tips for maximizing batch cooking:

1. Select Versatile Recipes: Make sure your recipe selections can be readily expanded to make a variety of dishes. For instance, you can use grilled chicken all week long in salads, wraps, and pasta meals.

2. Cook in Big Amounts: Make a lot of basic ingredients, such as grains, proteins, and roasted veggies. Divide them into portions and keep them chilled or frozen for easy assembling at a later time.

3. Use Multi-Functional Appliances: You can cook several things at once by using appliances like ovens, pressure cookers, and slow cookers. In the kitchen, this can save time and energy.

4. Proper Storage: Separate cooked food into serving portions and keep it in sealed containers. To keep track of what you have and prevent waste, label with the contents and the date.

Optimizing the Utilization of Ingredients

It is more cost-effective and environmentally responsible to minimize food waste and maximize ingredient utilization. The following are some tactics:

1. Try New Recipes: To keep your meals interesting and varied, try new recipes and cuisines on a regular basis. You may find new favorite recipes and ingredients this way as well.

2. Seasonal Ingredients: Include produce that is in season in your meal plans. Seasonal ingredients can be more economical in addition to being fresher and tastier.

3. Theme Nights: To give your weekly meal plan a fun twist, introduce theme nights like "Taco Tuesday" or "Stir-Fry Friday." Meal planning may become more fun and easy as a result.

4. Include Friends and Family: Involve your friends or family in the meal preparation process. In addition to being enjoyable and fulfilling, cooking together can help divide the workload.

Maintaining Consistency and Motivation

The secret to a successful meal prep is consistency. The following advice will help you stay inspired and stick to your meal prep schedule:

1. Establish Realistic Goals: Begin with attainable objectives and, as you gain comfort, progressively increase the complexity of your meal preparation schedule. This guarantees long-term success and avoids overwhelm.

2. Monitor Your Progress: Use a meal planning app or keep a meal prep journal to keep track of your progress, identify areas for improvement, and note what works well. Taking stock of your accomplishments can help you stay motivated.

3. Reward Yourself: When you reach your meal prep objectives, treat yourself to something fun. This could be an indulgent treat, a novel culinary tool, or a soothing pastime.

4. Remain Adaptable: Show flexibility and receptivity to change. Don't be scared to modify your meal prep schedule if something isn't working. You can discover what suits your lifestyle the best when you are flexible.

You can develop a gratifying and long-lasting habit that promotes your wellness and health objectives by implementing these pointers and techniques into your meal preparation routine. Key elements of a successful meal prep include keeping meals interesting, cooking in bulk, organizing the kitchen efficiently, and maintaining motivation. To ensure that everyone can benefit from meal prep, we'll discuss how to modify your meal prep for unique dietary requirements and preferences in the upcoming chapter. Cheers to your preparation!

CHAPTER TEN

Meal Preps for Special Occasions

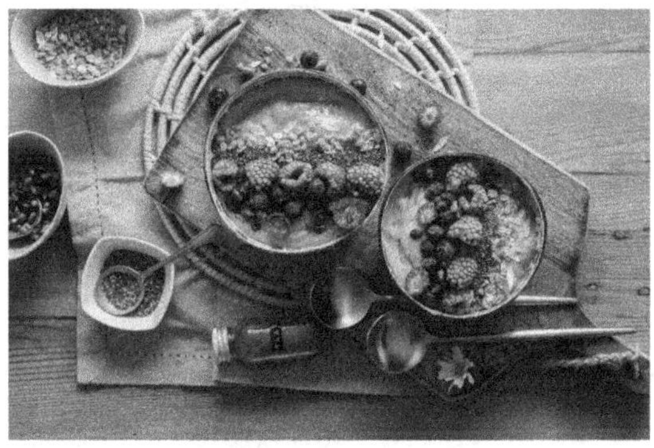

Not only can meal prep save lives on regular days, but it can also be a huge help during festivities and special occasions. Whether you're attending a potluck, throwing a dinner party, or celebrating a holiday, organizing and preparing ahead of time can help you save time, lower your stress level, and wow your guests with tasty food. We'll look at meal prep techniques and recipes in this chapter for a variety of special occasions so you can celebrate life's special moments without having to spend it in the kitchen.

Dinner Parties Simplified

Organizing a dinner party can be fun, but if you don't plan ahead, it can also be stressful. Here's how to simplify the preparation of dinner for guests:

1. Prepare Your Menu in Advance: Select the cuisine or theme for your dinner party and arrange your menu appropriately. Choose a variety of appetizers, main courses, side dishes, and desserts that go well together and are prepatable ahead of time.

2.Prepare Your Ingredients in Advance: Preparing ingredients in advance can help to speed up the cooking process the day of the party. Cut up vegetables, marinate meats, and make dressings and sauces. When you're ready to cook, keep prepared ingredients chilled in the fridge.

3. Choose Prepare-Ahead Meals: Select recipes that can be assembled right before serving or that can be prepared ahead of time and reheated. Delicious options that taste even better the next day include lasagnas, casseroles, and braised foods.

4. Set Up a Self-Serve Bar: Provide a selection of drinks, mixers, and garnishes for guests to help themselves from the bar during the evening. Your time can now be better spent on other aspects of hosting as a result.

5. Assign Tasks: Asking friends or family for assistance with meal preparation, table setting, or drink serving is nothing to be ashamed of. You may interact with your guests and enjoy the celebration by assigning tasks to others.

Simple Holiday Feasts

Although it's a time to celebrate, holiday get-togethers can also be stressful because there are lots of dishes to prepare. Here's how to prepare holiday meals more quickly:

1. Establish a Detailed Timetable: Arrange your cooking schedule and specify the times at which each dish should be ready and heated. This guarantees everything is ready on time and helps avoid rushing at the last minute.

2. Prepare the Make-Ahead Side Dishes: Select side dishes that are ready to eat and can be reheated right before the meal. Traditional holiday sides include roasted vegetables, stuffing, and mashed potatoes, all of which can be made ahead.

3. Make Use of Your Instant Pot and Slow Cooker:
Use slow cookers and Instant Pots to quickly prepare main courses such as roast beef, ham, or turkey. These gadgets keep food warm until serving time and free up oven space.

4. Provide a Range of Desserts: Make a few different desserts to accommodate dietary restrictions and a variety of tastes. Your guests will be delighted by traditional holiday desserts like pies, cakes, cookies, and festive treats.

5. Prepare a Festive Drink Station: Put together a festive drink station with seasonal concoctions like hot chocolate, spiked cider, and mulled wine. Give guests a selection of garnishes and mix-ins to personalize their drinks.

Perfect Potluck

Potlucks are an excellent method to distribute the workload and try different foods without placing all the burden on the host. How to make your potluck contribution shine:

1. Select a Dish That Will Please Many People:
Choose a dish, such as salads, dips, casseroles, or finger foods, that is portable and can be served at room temperature. When selecting your dish, take

into account the dietary requirements and preferences of your other guests.

2. Prepare the Ingredients in a Transportable Container: Gather the ingredients in a container that will be easy to carry to the potluck location. Steer clear of dishes that call for intricate presentation or last-minute assembly.

3. Label Your Food: Write your name and an ingredient list on the label, particularly if the dish includes any common allergens. This assists visitors with dietary requirements in finding suitable options.

4. Choose a Recipe That Will Appeal to a Wide Range of Audiences: Pick an appetizer that can be served at room temperature and is portable, like salads, dips, casseroles, or finger foods. Think about your other guests' dietary needs and preferences when choosing your dish.

5. Arrange the Components into a Conveyable Container: Put the ingredients in a carry-friendly container and head to the potluck location. Avoid recipes that require complicated assembly or last-minute presentation.

6. Label Your Food: Include a list of ingredients and your name on the label, especially if the dish contains any common allergens. This helps guests with special dietary needs locate appropriate options.

Conclusion

When it comes to special occasions, meal prep can make all the difference. It liberates you from the burden of last-minute cooking so you can enjoy unforgettable get-togethers with friends and family. Cooking ahead of time will enable you to produce mouthwatering dishes that will wow your guests and leave a lasting impression, whether you're throwing a dinner party, attending a potluck, or celebrating a holiday. This chapter contains recipes and advice that will help you prepare for any special occasion and make it easy to handle. Too many happy years of entertainment and festivities!

DAILY MEAL REMARK

DAYS	RECIPES	REMARKS

www.ingramcontent.com/pod-product-compliance
Lightning Source LLC
Chambersburg PA
CBHW072337270726
48659CB00022B/1836

1. In una piccola ciotola, mescolate lo zucchero di canna e il miele fino a ottenere una pasta granulosa.

2. Se lo desiderate, potete aggiungere un cucchiaino di olio di cocco per un'idratazione extra.

3. Applicate lo scrub sulle labbra asciutte e pulite.

4. Massaggiate delicatamente con movimenti circolari per alcuni minuti per esfoliare le labbra e rimuovere le cellule morte.

5. Risciacquate con acqua tiepida e tamponate le labbra asciutte.

Benefici: Lo zucchero di canna agisce come un'esfoliante naturale, eliminando delicatamente le cellule morte e rendendo le labbra più lisce e levigate. Il miele è noto per le sue proprietà idratanti e lenitive, che aiutano a mantenere le labbra morbide e idratate. L'olio di cocco aggiunge un ulteriore strato di idratazione, lasciando le labbra nutrienti e protette dall'essiccazione.

Questo scrub labbra fai-da-te è un modo semplice e efficace per mantenere le labbra morbide e lisce tutto l'anno. Integrate questo trattamento nella vostra routine di bellezza e preparatevi a mostrare un sorriso radioso e irresistibile.

Capitolo 7: Olio detergente all'olio di mandorle dolci La pulizia della pelle è fondamentale per mantenere un aspetto sano e luminoso. In questo capitolo, esploreremo come preparare un delicato olio detergente utilizzando l'olio di mandorle dolci, perfetto per rimuovere il trucco e le impurità senza compromettere l'idratazione della pelle.

Ingredienti:

• 2 cucchiai di olio di mandorle dolci

• 1 cucchiaio di olio di jojoba (opzionale)

• 2 gocce di olio essenziale di lavanda (opzionale) **Istruzioni:**

1. In una piccola bottiglia, versate l'olio di mandorle dolci.

2. Se lo desiderate, aggiungete l'olio di jojoba per un'azione detergente ancora più efficace.

3. Aggiungete alcune gocce di olio essenziale di lavanda per un profumo rilassante e lenitivo.

4. Chiudete la bottiglia e agitatela delicatamente per miscelare gli ingredienti.

Modo d'uso:

1. Versate una piccola quantità di olio detergente sulla pelle asciutta del viso.

2. Massaggiate delicatamente con movimenti circolari per un paio di minuti, concentrando l'attenzione sulle aree in cui si accumula il trucco.

3. Bagnate un batuffolo di cotone con acqua tiepida e utilizzatelo per rimuovere l'olio e il trucco.

4. Risciacquate il viso con acqua tiepida e tamponate delicatamente con un asciugamano.

Benefici: L'olio di mandorle dolci è ricco di vitamine e antiossidanti che nutrono e idratano la pelle, lasciandola morbida e levigata. L'olio di jojoba è simile al sebo prodotto naturalmente dalla pelle e può aiutare a regolare la produzione di sebo, mantenendo la pelle equilibrata e priva di impurità. L'olio essenziale di lavanda aggiunge un tocco di freschezza e contribuisce a lenire la pelle irritata o sensibile.

Questo olio detergente all'olio di mandorle dolci è ideale per tutti i tipi di pelle, anche per quelli più sensibili. Aggiungetelo alla vostra routine di pulizia quotidiana e godetevi una pelle pulita, morbida e luminosa.

Capitolo 8: Tonico al cetriolo

Il cetriolo è noto per le sue proprietà lenitive e idratanti, rendendolo un ingrediente ideale per un tonico rigenerante per la pelle. In questo capitolo, vi mostrerò come preparare un tonico rinfrescante che calma e tonifica la pelle, lasciandola radiosa e rivitalizzata.

Ingredienti:

• 1 cetriolo medio

• ½ tazza di acqua di rose

• 1 cucchiaino di succo di limone (opzionale)

Istruzioni:

1. Tagliate il cetriolo a fette sottili e mettetelo in un frullatore.

2. Frullate il cetriolo fino a ottenere una consistenza liscia e omogenea.

3. Utilizzate un colino o un telo di cotone per filtrare il succo di cetriolo in una ciotola.

4. Aggiungete l'acqua di rose al succo di cetriolo e mescolate bene.

5. Se lo desiderate, potete aggiungere un cucchiaino di succo di limone per un'azione tonificante extra.

6. Trasferite il tonico in una bottiglia spray e conservatelo in frigorifero per mantenerlo fresco.

Modo d'uso:

1. Dopo aver detergente il viso, chiudete gli occhi e spruzzate il tonico sulla pelle.

2. Tamponate delicatamente con un batuffolo di cotone per distribuirlo uniformemente.

3. Lasciate asciugare naturalmente o tamponate leggermente con un asciugamano morbido.

4. Applicate la crema idratante abituale per completare la vostra routine di cura della pelle.

Benefici: Il cetriolo è ricco di acqua e nutrienti essenziali che idratano e leniscono la pelle, riducendo il rossore e il gonfiore. L'acqua di rose ha proprietà tonificanti e rinfrescanti, mentre il succo di limone può contribuire a ridurre l'aspetto dei pori e a illuminare la pelle. Insieme, questi ingredienti creano un tonico che rivitalizza e rinfresca la pelle, lasciandola luminosa, tonica e radiosa.

Aggiungete questo tonico al cetriolo alla vostra routine di bellezza quotidiana e godetevi i benefici della sua azione lenitiva e tonificante per una pelle sana e luminosa.

Capitolo 9: Maschera al miele e cannella La combinazione di miele e cannella crea una maschera potente con numerosi benefici per la pelle, dalla riduzione dell'infiammazione all'azione antibatterica. In questo capitolo, vi guiderò nella preparazione di questa maschera rigenerante, perfetta per combattere l'acne e migliorare l'aspetto della pelle.

Ingredienti:

• 2 cucchiai di miele

• 1 cucchiaino di cannella in polvere

• ½ cucchiaino di succo di limone (opzionale)

Istruzioni:

1. In una ciotola, mescolate il miele e la cannella fino a ottenere una pasta densa e omogenea.

2. Se lo desiderate, potete aggiungere un cucchiaino di succo di limone per un'azione esfoliante e schiarente.

3. Applicate uniformemente la maschera sulla pelle pulita e asciutta del viso, evitando il contorno occhi e labbra.

4. Lasciate agire per circa 10-15 minuti.

5. Risciacquate abbondantemente con acqua tiepida e tamponate delicatamente per asciugare.

Benefici: Il miele è noto per le sue proprietà antibatteriche e idratanti, che aiutano a ridurre l'infiammazione e a mantenere la pelle morbida e luminosa. La cannella è ricca di antiossidanti e ha proprietà antinfiammatorie, che possono aiutare a combattere l'acne e a ridurre i rossori. Il succo di limone contiene acidi alfa idrossi che esfoliano delicatamente la pelle, riducendo l'aspetto delle imperfezioni e delle macchie scure.

Questa maschera al miele e cannella è un trattamento efficace per migliorare la texture della pelle e combattere l'acne in modo naturale. Integrate questa maschera nella vostra routine di cura della pelle e preparatevi a godere dei benefici di una pelle più chiara, luminosa e priva di imperfezioni.

Capitolo 10: Impacco per capelli all'avocado L'avocado è un frutto ricco di nutrienti che può trasformare i capelli secchi e danneggiati in chiome morbide e lucenti. In questo capitolo, vi mostrerò come preparare un impacco nutriente utilizzando l'avocado come ingrediente principale.

Ingredienti:

• 1 avocado maturo

• 2 cucchiai di olio di cocco

• 1 tuorlo d'uovo (opzionale)

Istruzioni:

1. In una ciotola, schiacciate l'avocado fino a ottenere una consistenza cremosa e priva di grumi.

2. Aggiungete l'olio di cocco e mescolate bene fino a ottenere un composto omogeneo.

3. Se lo desiderate, potete aggiungere un tuorlo d'uovo per un'idratazione extra e per rinforzare i capelli.

4. Applicate l'impacco sui capelli asciutti, concentrando l'attenzione sulle lunghezze e sulle punte.

5. Massaggiate delicatamente il cuoio capelluto per favorire l'assorbimento dei nutrienti.

6. Avvolgete i capelli con una cuffia da doccia o della pellicola trasparente e lasciate in posa per almeno 30 minuti.

7. Dopo il tempo di posa, lavate i capelli con il vostro shampoo abituale e risciacquate bene.

Benefici: L'avocado è ricco di grassi naturali, vitamine e minerali che idratano e nutrono i capelli, riparando i danni e migliorandone la lucentezza e la morbidezza. L'olio di cocco penetra nel fusto del capello, fornendo idratazione e protezione dai danni ambientali. Il tuorlo d'uovo è ricco di proteine che rinforzano i capelli e ne migliorano la struttura.

Questo impacco all'avocado è un trattamento lussuoso che trasforma istantaneamente i capelli secchi e danneggiati in una chioma radiosa e sana. Utilizzatelo regolarmente per mantenere i vostri capelli morbidi, lucenti e pieni di vitalità.

Capitolo 11: Scrub corpo al sale marino Il sale marino è un eccellente esfoliante naturale che può aiutare a rimuovere le cellule morte dalla pelle, lasciandola morbida, liscia e luminosa. In questo capitolo, vi mostrerò come preparare uno scrub corpo rigenerante utilizzando il sale marino e altri ingredienti nutrienti.

Ingredienti:

• 1 tazza di sale marino grosso

• ½ tazza di olio di cocco

• 10 gocce di olio essenziale di arancia dolce (opzionale)
Istruzioni:

1. In una ciotola, mescolate il sale marino grosso con l'olio di cocco fino a ottenere una consistenza granulosa e umida.

2. Se lo desiderate, potete aggiungere alcune gocce di olio essenziale di arancia dolce per un profumo fresco e rivitalizzante.

3. Applicate lo scrub sulla pelle umida durante la doccia o il bagno, concentrando l'attenzione sulle aree ruvide o secche.

4. Massaggiate delicatamente con movimenti circolari per alcuni minuti, quindi risciacquate abbondantemente con acqua tiepida.

5. Tamponate delicatamente la pelle con un asciugamano per asciugarla.

Benefici: Il sale marino agisce come un'esfoliante naturale, rimuovendo le cellule morte dalla superficie della pelle e migliorandone la texture. L'olio di cocco idrata e nutre la pelle in profondità, lasciandola morbida e luminosa. L'olio essenziale di arancia dolce aggiunge un profumo fresco e vivace, mentre le sue proprietà stimolanti contribuiscono a ravvivare la pelle stanca e spenta.

Questo scrub corpo al sale marino è un trattamento lussuoso che lascia la vostra pelle radiosa, levigata e profumata. Utilizzatelo una o due volte a settimana per mantenere la vostra pelle morbida, liscia e luminosa tutto l'anno.

Capitolo 12: Maschera viso all'avena e miele L'avena è conosciuta per le sue proprietà lenitive e idratanti, mentre il miele è un potente agente idratante e antibatterico. In questo capitolo, vi guiderò nella preparazione di una maschera viso rigenerante che combina questi due ingredienti per una pelle luminosa e idratata.

Ingredienti:

• 2 cucchiai di fiocchi d'avena

• 1 cucchiaio di miele

• 1-2 cucchiai di acqua (o latte vegetale)

Istruzioni:

1. In una ciotola, versate i fiocchi d'avena e schiacciateli leggermente con un cucchiaio per ottenere una consistenza più fine.

2. Aggiungete il miele e mescolate bene fino a ottenere un composto omogeneo.

3. Aggiungete gradualmente l'acqua o il latte vegetale fino a ottenere una pasta spalmabile.

4. Applicate la maschera uniformemente sul viso, evitando il contorno occhi.

5. Lasciate agire per circa 10-15 minuti.

6. Risciacquate abbondantemente con acqua tiepida e tamponate delicatamente per asciugare.

Benefici: L'avena è ricca di antiossidanti e beta-glucani che leniscono la pelle irritata e riducono l'infiammazione. Il miele ha proprietà idratanti, antibatteriche e antinfiammatorie, che aiutano a mantenere la pelle morbida, pulita e luminosa. Insieme, questi ingredienti creano una maschera viso che idrata in profondità, lenisce le irritazioni e dona alla pelle un aspetto fresco e radioso.

Questa maschera all'avena e miele è adatta a tutti i tipi di pelle, anche a quelle più sensibili.

Utilizzatela una o due volte a settimana per mantenere la vostra pelle idratata, luminosa e visibilmente più giovane.

Capitolo 13: Balsamo labbra al burro di cacao e olio di mandorle Le labbra hanno bisogno di idratazione e protezione, specialmente durante i mesi più freddi o secchi dell'anno. In questo capitolo, vi mostrerò come preparare un balsamo labbra rigenerante utilizzando il burro di cacao e l'olio di mandorle, ingredienti naturali ricchi di proprietà nutrienti.

Ingredienti:

• 1 cucchiaio di burro di cacao

• 1 cucchiaio di olio di mandorle dolci

• 1 cucchiaino di cera d'api (opzionale per una consistenza più solida)

• 2 gocce di olio essenziale di vaniglia (opzionale per un aroma delizioso) **Istruzioni:**

1. In un pentolino a bagnomaria, fate sciogliere il burro di cacao e l'olio di mandorle dolci a fuoco basso, mescolando delicatamente finché non si saranno completamente fusi.

2. Se desiderate una consistenza più solida per il vostro balsamo, aggiungete la cera d'api e mescolate finché non si sarà completamente sciolta.

3. Rimuovete dal fuoco e lasciate raffreddare leggermente.

4. Aggiungete l'olio essenziale di vaniglia per un aroma delizioso e mescolate bene.

5. Versate il composto in piccoli contenitori o barattolini puliti e sterilizzati.

6. Lasciate raffreddare completamente a temperatura ambiente fino a quando il balsamo non sarà solido.

Modo d'uso:

1. Applicate una piccola quantità di balsamo sulle labbra secondo necessità, soprattutto quando sono secche o screpolate.

2. Massaggiate delicatamente per far assorbire il balsamo.

Benefici: Il burro di cacao è ricco di antiossidanti e acidi grassi che idratano e riparano le labbra secche e danneggiate. L'olio di mandorle dolci penetra nella pelle, fornendo idratazione e nutrimento. La cera d'api aggiunge una consistenza solida al balsamo e crea una barriera protettiva sulla superficie delle labbra. L'olio essenziale di vaniglia aggiunge un aroma delizioso e contribuisce a lenire le labbra secche.

Questo balsamo labbra fatto in casa è una soluzione naturale per mantenere le labbra morbide, idratate e protette dagli agenti atmosferici. Utilizzatelo regolarmente per labbra sempre belle e curate.

Capitolo 14: Maschera per il viso al cetriolo e yogurt Il cetriolo è noto per le sue proprietà idratanti e lenitive, mentre lo yogurt è ricco di enzimi e acidi lattici che aiutano a esfoliare e levigare la pelle. In questo capitolo, vi guiderò nella preparazione di una maschera viso rigenerante che combina questi due ingredienti per una pelle fresca e luminosa.

Ingredienti:

• ½ cetriolo

• 2 cucchiai di yogurt naturale

Istruzioni:

1. Sbucciate il cetriolo e tagliatelo a fette sottili.

2. Mettete le fette di cetriolo in un frullatore e frullatele fino a ottenere una consistenza liscia.

3. Trasferite il cetriolo frullato in una ciotola e aggiungete lo yogurt.

4. Mescolate bene fino a ottenere un composto omogeneo.

Modo d'uso:

1. Dopo aver detergente il viso, applicate uniformemente la maschera sul viso e sul collo, evitando il contorno occhi.

2. Lasciate agire per circa 15-20 minuti.

3. Risciacquate abbondantemente con acqua tiepida e tamponate delicatamente per asciugare.

Benefici: Il cetriolo è ricco di acqua e nutrienti che idratano e leniscono la pelle, riducendo il rossore e il gonfiore. Lo yogurt contiene acidi lattici che esfoliano delicatamente la pelle, rimuovendo le cellule morte e migliorandone la texture. Insieme, questi ingredienti creano una maschera viso che idrata, lenisce e rinfresca la pelle, lasciandola luminosa e rivitalizzata.

Utilizzate questa maschera al cetriolo e yogurt una o due volte a settimana per mantenere la vostra pelle idratata, luminosa e visibilmente più giovane.

Capitolo 15: Scrub corpo al caffè e olio di cocco Il caffè non è solo un ottimo stimolante per il mattino, ma può anche essere un efficace esfoliante per la pelle. In questo capitolo, vi mostrerò come preparare uno scrub corpo rigenerante utilizzando il caffè e l'olio di cocco, perfetto per rivitalizzare e tonificare la pelle.

Ingredienti:

• 1 tazza di caffè macinato

• ½ tazza di olio di cocco

• 2 cucchiai di zucchero di canna (opzionale per un'esfoliazione extra) **Istruzioni:**

1. In una ciotola, mescolate il caffè macinato con l'olio di cocco fino a ottenere una consistenza granulosa.

2. Se desiderate un'esfoliazione extra, aggiungete anche lo zucchero di canna e mescolate bene.

3. Applicate lo scrub sulla pelle umida durante la doccia o il bagno, concentrando l'attenzione sulle aree ruvide o secche.

4. Massaggiate delicatamente con movimenti circolari per alcuni minuti, quindi risciacquate abbondantemente con acqua tiepida.

5. Tamponate delicatamente la pelle con un asciugamano per asciugarla.

Benefici: Il caffè contiene caffeina e antiossidanti che stimolano la circolazione sanguigna e riducono l'aspetto della cellulite e delle smagliature. L'olio di cocco idrata e nutre la pelle in profondità, lasciandola morbida e luminosa. Lo zucchero di canna agisce come un'esfoliante naturale, rimuovendo le cellule morte dalla superficie della pelle e migliorandone la texture.

Utilizzate questo scrub corpo al caffè e olio di cocco una o due volte a settimana per mantenere la vostra pelle morbida, liscia e luminosa, e per godere dei benefici stimolanti e tonificanti del caffè.

Capitolo 16: Maschera per capelli alla banana e miele La banana è ricca di vitamine, minerali e oli naturali che possono idratare e rinforzare i capelli danneggiati. In questo capitolo, vi guiderò nella preparazione di una maschera per capelli fai-da-te utilizzando la banana e il miele, per ottenere una chioma morbida, lucente e nutrita.

Ingredienti:

• 1 banana matura

• 2 cucchiai di miele

• 1 cucchiaio di olio di cocco (opzionale per capelli molto secchi)
Istruzioni:

1. Sbucciate la banana e tagliatela a pezzi.

2. Mettete i pezzi di banana in una ciotola e schiacciateli con una forchetta fino a ottenere una consistenza cremosa e priva di grumi.

3. Aggiungete il miele e mescolate bene fino a ottenere un composto omogeneo.

4. Se i vostri capelli sono particolarmente secchi, potete aggiungere anche un cucchiaio di olio di cocco e mescolare bene.

5. Applicate la maschera sui capelli asciutti, concentrandovi sulle lunghezze e sulle punte.

6. Massaggiate delicatamente il cuoio capelluto per favorire l'assorbimento dei nutrienti.

7. Avvolgete i capelli con una cuffia da doccia o della pellicola trasparente e lasciate in posa per almeno 30 minuti.

8. Dopo il tempo di posa, lavate i capelli con il vostro shampoo abituale e risciacquate bene.

Benefici: La banana è ricca di potassio, vitamine e oli naturali che possono nutrire, idratare e rinforzare i capelli, riducendo la secchezza e la fragilità. Il miele è un potente idratante e ammorbidente che può aggiungere lucentezza e morbidezza ai capelli. L'olio di cocco penetra nel fusto del capello, fornendo idratazione e protezione dai danni ambientali.

Questa maschera per capelli alla banana e miele è un trattamento lussuoso che trasforma i capelli secchi e danneggiati in una chioma morbida, lucente e piena di vitalità. Utilizzatela regolarmente per mantenere i vostri capelli sani e belli.

Capitolo 17: Esfoliante labbra al miele e zucchero di canna Le labbra hanno bisogno di cure speciali per rimanere morbide e lisce, soprattutto durante i mesi più freddi o secchi dell'anno. In questo capitolo, vi mostrerò come preparare un esfoliante labbra fai-da-te utilizzando il miele e lo zucchero di canna, per eliminare le cellule morte e ottenere labbra vellutate e morbide.

Ingredienti:

• 1 cucchiaino di miele

• 1 cucchiaino di zucchero di canna

Istruzioni:

1. In una piccola ciotola, mescolate il miele con lo zucchero di canna fino a ottenere una pasta granulosa.

2. Assicuratevi che gli ingredienti siano ben combinati per formare una consistenza omogenea.

Modo d'uso:

1. Applicate una piccola quantità di esfoliante sulle labbra asciutte e pulite.

2. Massaggiate delicatamente con movimenti circolari per un paio di minuti, concentrando l'attenzione sulle aree secche o ruvide.

3. Risciacquate abbondantemente con acqua tiepida e tamponate delicatamente per asciugare.

4. Applicate quindi un balsamo labbra idratante per completare il trattamento.

Benefici: Il miele è un potente idratante naturale che ammorbidisce e lenisce le labbra secche, mentre lo zucchero di canna agisce come un'esfoliante delicato, rimuovendo le cellule morte e migliorando la texture delle labbra. Insieme, questi ingredienti creano un esfoliante labbra efficace che le lascia morbide, lisce e vellutate.

Utilizzate questo esfoliante labbra al miele e zucchero di canna una o due volte a settimana per mantenere le vostre labbra morbide, lisce e visibilmente più belle.

Capitolo 18: Maschera al cetriolo e yogurt per il viso Il cetriolo è rinomato per le sue proprietà lenitive e rinfrescanti sulla pelle, mentre lo yogurt è ricco di enzimi che possono esfoliare delicatamente e idratare. In questo capitolo, vi guiderò nella preparazione di una maschera viso fai-da-te utilizzando cetriolo e yogurt, per una pelle rinfrescata e luminosa.

Ingredienti:

• ½ cetriolo

• 2 cucchiai di yogurt naturale

Istruzioni:

1. Sbucciate il cetriolo e tagliatelo a pezzetti.

2. Mettete i pezzi di cetriolo e lo yogurt in un frullatore.

3. Frullate fino a ottenere un composto liscio e omogeneo.

4. Trasferite la miscela in una ciotola.

Modo d'uso:

1. Dopo aver detergente il viso, applicate uniformemente la maschera sul viso e sul collo, evitando il contorno occhi.

2. Lasciate agire per circa 15-20 minuti.

3. Risciacquate abbondantemente con acqua tiepida e tamponate delicatamente per asciugare.

Benefici: Il cetriolo è composto principalmente da acqua, che idrata e lenisce la pelle, riducendo il rossore e il gonfiore. Lo yogurt contiene enzimi che possono esfoliare delicatamente la pelle, rimuovendo le cellule morte e migliorandone la texture. Insieme, questi ingredienti creano una maschera viso che rinfresca, idrata e ravviva la pelle, lasciandola luminosa e rivitalizzata.

Utilizzate questa maschera al cetriolo e yogurt una o due volte a settimana per mantenere la vostra pelle idratata, fresca e visibilmente più giovane.

Capitolo 19: Tonico al tea tree per pelli impure Il tea tree, o albero del tè, è noto per le sue proprietà antibatteriche e antinfiammatorie, ideali per contrastare l'acne e le imperfezioni della pelle. In questo capitolo, esploreremo la preparazione di un tonico naturale al tea tree, perfetto per detergere e purificare la pelle impura.

Ingredienti:

• 1 tazza di acqua

• 2-3 gocce di olio essenziale di tea tree

Istruzioni:

1. Portate l'acqua ad ebollizione in una pentola.

2. Una volta raggiunto il punto di ebollizione, rimuovete la pentola dal fuoco e lasciate raffreddare per alcuni minuti.

3. Aggiungete le gocce di olio essenziale di tea tree all'acqua e mescolate bene.

4. Trasferite il tonico in una bottiglia spray pulita e sterilizzata.

Modo d'uso:

1. Dopo aver detergente il viso, chiudete gli occhi e spruzzate il tonico sulla pelle.

2. Tamponate delicatamente con un batuffolo di cotone per distribuirlo uniformemente.

3. Lasciate asciugare naturalmente o tamponate leggermente con un asciugamano morbido.

4. Applicate la crema idratante abituale per completare la vostra routine di cura della pelle.

Benefici: L'olio essenziale di tea tree ha potenti proprietà antibatteriche e antinfiammatorie che possono aiutare a combattere l'acne e a ridurre l'infiammazione della pelle. Utilizzato come tonico, aiuta a detergere i pori in profondità e a purificare la pelle, riducendo la comparsa di imperfezioni e punti neri. Inoltre, il tea tree ha un effetto rinfrescante e lenitivo sulla pelle, lasciandola pulita, tonica e luminosa.

Questo tonico al tea tree è particolarmente indicato per le pelli impure e acneiche. Utilizzatelo regolarmente per mantenere la vostra pelle chiara, pulita e priva di imperfezioni.

Capitolo 20: Maschera lenitiva all'aloe vera e cetriolo L'aloe vera è rinomata per le sue proprietà lenitive e idratanti, mentre il cetriolo è noto per il suo effetto rinfrescante e rigenerante sulla pelle. In questo capitolo, esploreremo la preparazione di una maschera lenitiva che combina questi due ingredienti, perfetta per calmare la pelle irritata e ridare freschezza al viso.

Ingredienti:

• 2 cucchiai di gel di aloe vera

• ¼ di cetriolo

• 1 cucchiaino di succo di limone (opzionale per un effetto schiarente) **Istruzioni:**

1. Sbucciate il cetriolo e tagliatelo a pezzi.

2. Mettete i pezzi di cetriolo in un frullatore e frullateli fino a ottenere una consistenza liscia.

3. Trasferite il purè di cetriolo in una ciotola e aggiungete il gel di aloe vera.

4. Mescolate bene fino a ottenere un composto omogeneo.

5. Se lo desiderate, aggiungete il succo di limone e mescolate di nuovo.

Modo d'uso:

1. Dopo aver detergente il viso, applicate uniformemente la maschera sul viso e sul collo, evitando il contorno occhi.

2. Lasciate agire per circa 15-20 minuti.

3. Risciacquate abbondantemente con acqua tiepida e tamponate delicatamente per asciugare.

Benefici: Il gel di aloe vera ha proprietà lenitive e idratanti che possono ridurre l'infiammazione e calmare la pelle irritata o arrossata. Il cetriolo è ricco di acqua e nutrienti che idratano e rinfrescano la pelle, mentre il succo di limone può contribuire a schiarire le macchie scure e uniformare l'incarnato. Insieme, questi ingredienti creano una maschera lenitiva che ridona freschezza e luminosità alla pelle, lasciandola morbida e radiosa.

Utilizzate questa maschera all'aloe vera e cetriolo una o due volte a settimana per mantenere la vostra pelle calma, idratata e visibilmente più giovane.

Conclusione: Elevare la Bellezza Naturale con Rimedi Casalinghi Arrivati alla fine di questo viaggio attraverso le ricette e i segreti della bellezza fai-da-te, ci troviamo di fronte a un mondo di possibilità che si aprono nella nostra stessa cucina e dispensa.

Durante questo percorso, abbiamo esplorato un'ampia gamma di ingredienti naturali e semplici tecniche che possono trasformare la nostra routine di cura personale in un momento di benessere e auto-cura.

Le ricette presentate in questo libro non solo offrono soluzioni efficaci per migliorare l'aspetto della nostra pelle, dei nostri capelli e delle nostre labbra, ma ci invitano anche a riflettere sul concetto stesso di bellezza. Abbiamo imparato che la vera bellezza non risiede solo nell'aspetto esteriore, ma anche nell'attenzione e nell'amore che dedichiamo a noi stessi.

Ogni maschera, scrub e impacco per il corpo che abbiamo creato ci ha dato l'opportunità di prendere cura di noi stessi in modo consapevole, rispettando il nostro corpo e la natura che ci circonda. Abbiamo scoperto il potere di ingredienti semplici come il miele, l'avocado, il cetriolo e l'olio di cocco, che non solo nutrono la nostra pelle e i nostri capelli, ma ci collegano anche alle antiche tradizioni di cura della bellezza che risalgono a secoli fa.

Oltre a offrire benefici tangibili per la nostra bellezza esteriore, queste ricette ci incoraggiano anche a rallentare, a respirare profondamente e a dedicare del tempo a noi stessi in un mondo che spesso ci spinge ad andare sempre più veloce. Sono un invito a riconnetterci con il nostro corpo, ad ascoltarne i bisogni e a celebrarne la bellezza in tutte le sue forme.

Che tu abbia già sperimentato il piacere della creazione di rimedi casalinghi o che tu sia nuovo a questo mondo, spero che questo libro ti abbia ispirato a esplorare ulteriormente le infinite possibilità che la bellezza naturale offre. Che tu utilizzi queste ricette come parte della tua routine di cura personale quotidiana o che le riservi per un trattamento speciale, ricorda sempre che la bellezza è un viaggio, non una destinazione, e che la tua bellezza naturale brilla più luminosa quando ti prendi cura di te stesso con amore e gentilezza.

Con questo, ti ringrazio per avermi accompagnato in questo viaggio e ti auguro una bellezza radiante, sia dentro che fuori.

Con amore,

JANETCL

www.ingramcontent.com/pod-product-compliance
Lightning Source LLC
Chambersburg PA
CBHW072346270726
48659CB00023B/2414